WHO WILL YOU BE?

DAWN BARRETT

ILLUSTRATED BY: HALEY BARRETT,
MARSHA PETTITT AND ALAN TEAGUE

DEDICATION

This book is dedicated to all the unborn children in the world who have special people waiting for their arrival! Especially, my third grandchild, –Lovingly called for now, Barrett 3.

ACKNOWLEDGEMENT

Thank you, to my precious husband and friend who believes in me and pushes me to use my God-given talents to encourage others; my children, their spouses, and grandchildren—I love you all—further than the moon, my siblings who are the best! My sounding boards, prayer partners, and friends, you know who you are! Most importantly, Jesus Christ for giving us the ultimate gift of life!

I ask myself over and over, "Who will you be?"

One thing is for sure, you're an answer to prayer, just for me!

I wonder at the miracles happening in the "secret place,"

I wish I could watch you growing at such a rapid, wonderful pace!

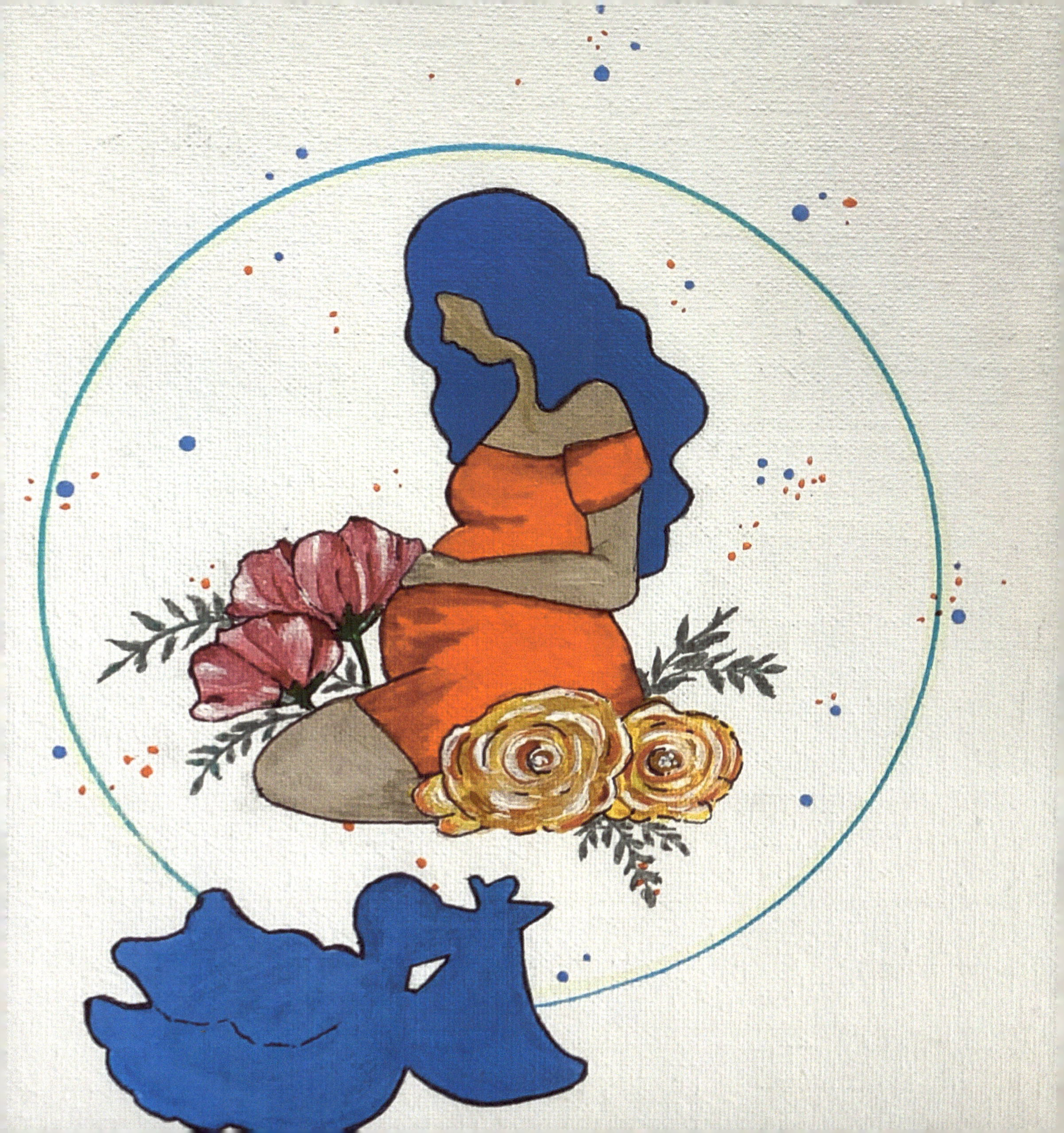

Around Week 5, you have blood cells & the beginnings of
your heart,
To our Creator, that just might be the most important part!
At Week 8, we can see your itsy, bitsy tiny hands and feet,
You are a miracle in the making, even though you are still
not complete!

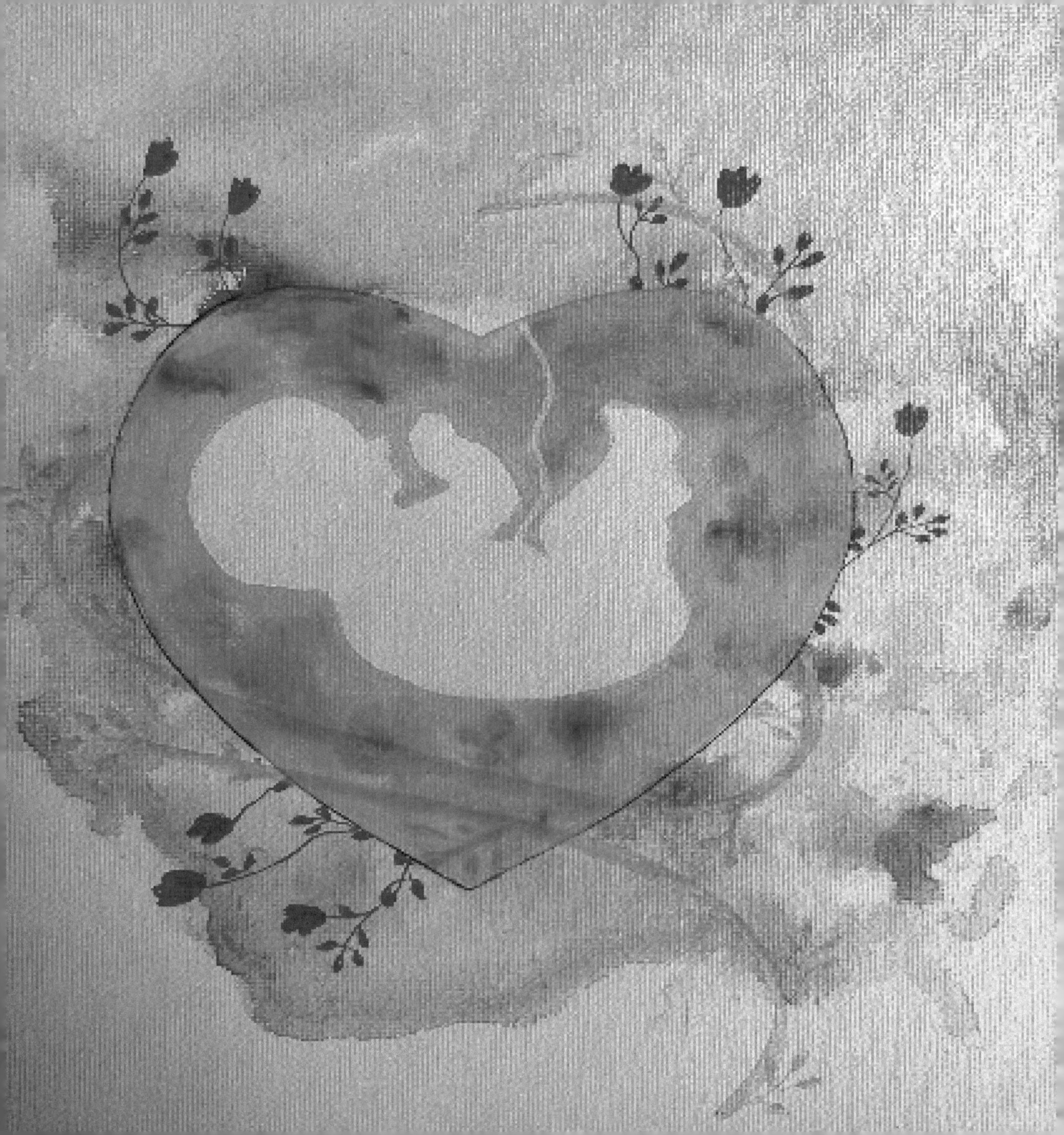

Will you be *Simon Gray, Sarah Louise* or maybe *Adam Rhett,*
We just don't know, can't know—will we ever know? Yes, just not YET!
You have eyelids around Week 10, and you can finally hear!
I love that where you are, you have absolutely nothing to fear!

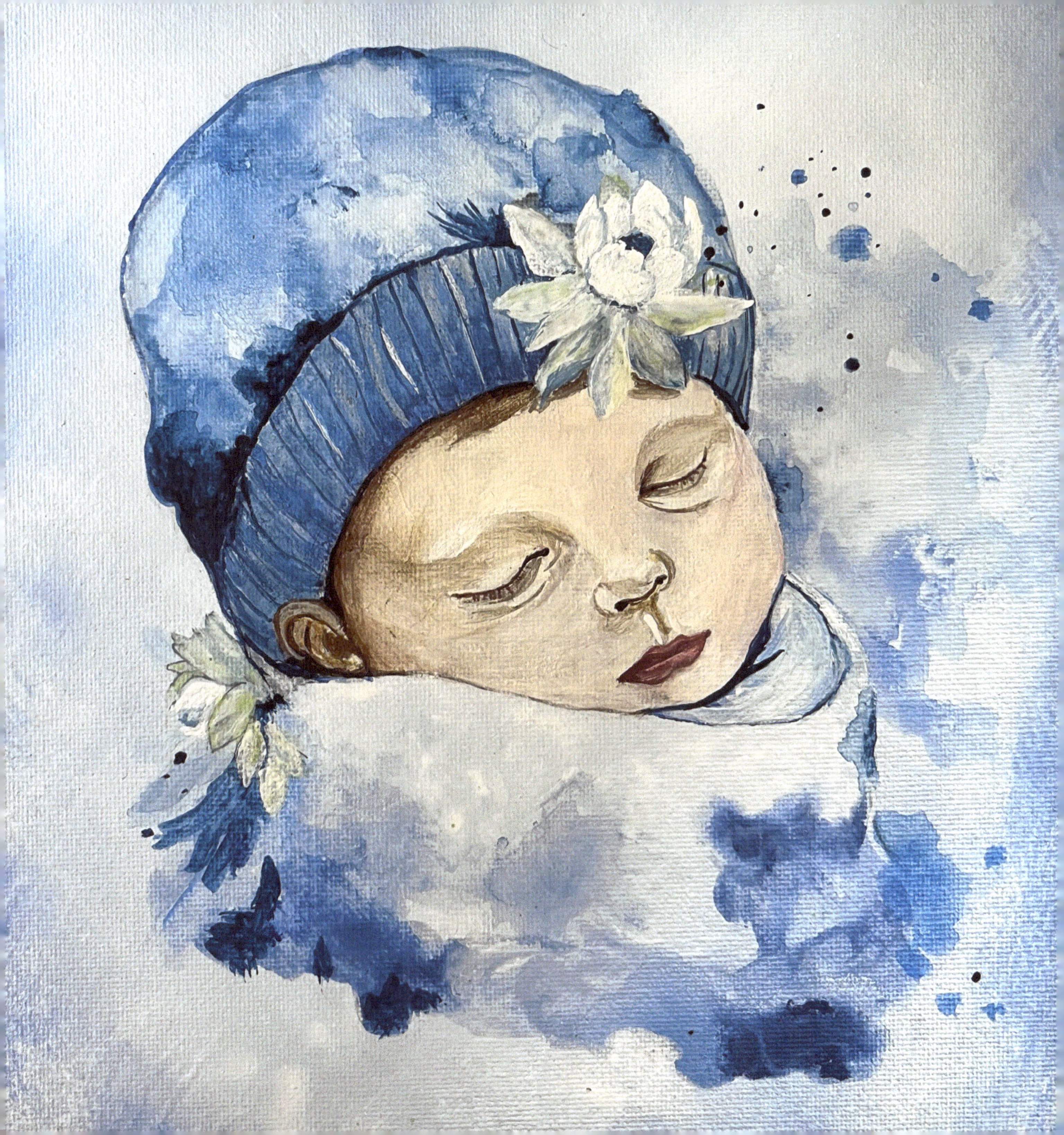

Between Weeks 11 & 14, you can make a fist & your face is delicate and smooth,
You kick and turn, flitter and flutter, and your mom is anxious to feel you move!
Will you be shy or outgoing, maybe a hunter like your dad?
Will you have a temper, or will it take a lot to make you mad?

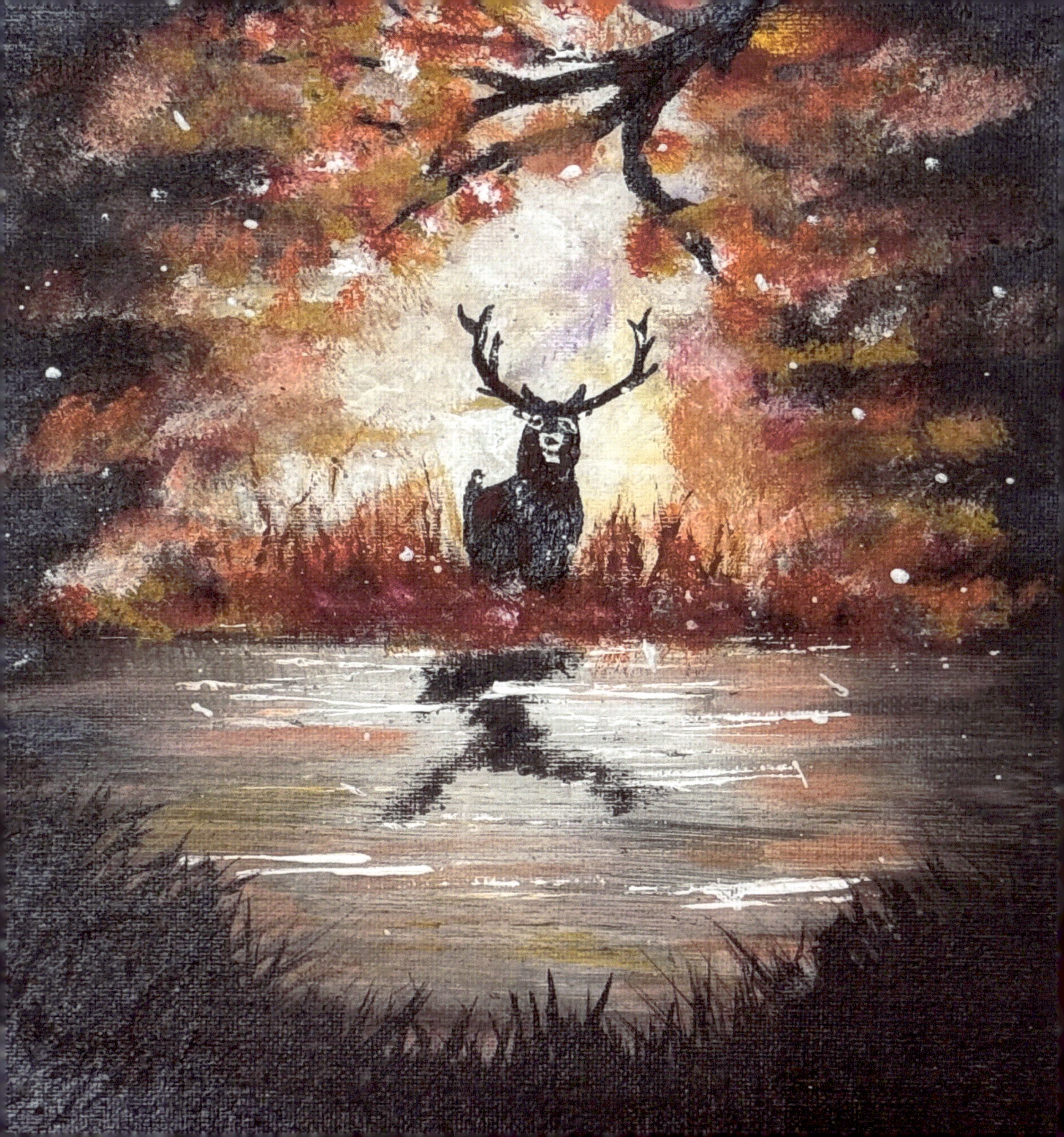

Who will you be, a gift straight from heaven for me?

Will you like cars, trucks, baby dolls or trees?

And what will your very favorite animal be?

Will your eyes be blue, or will they be brown?

Will you play in the country or dance a jig in the town?

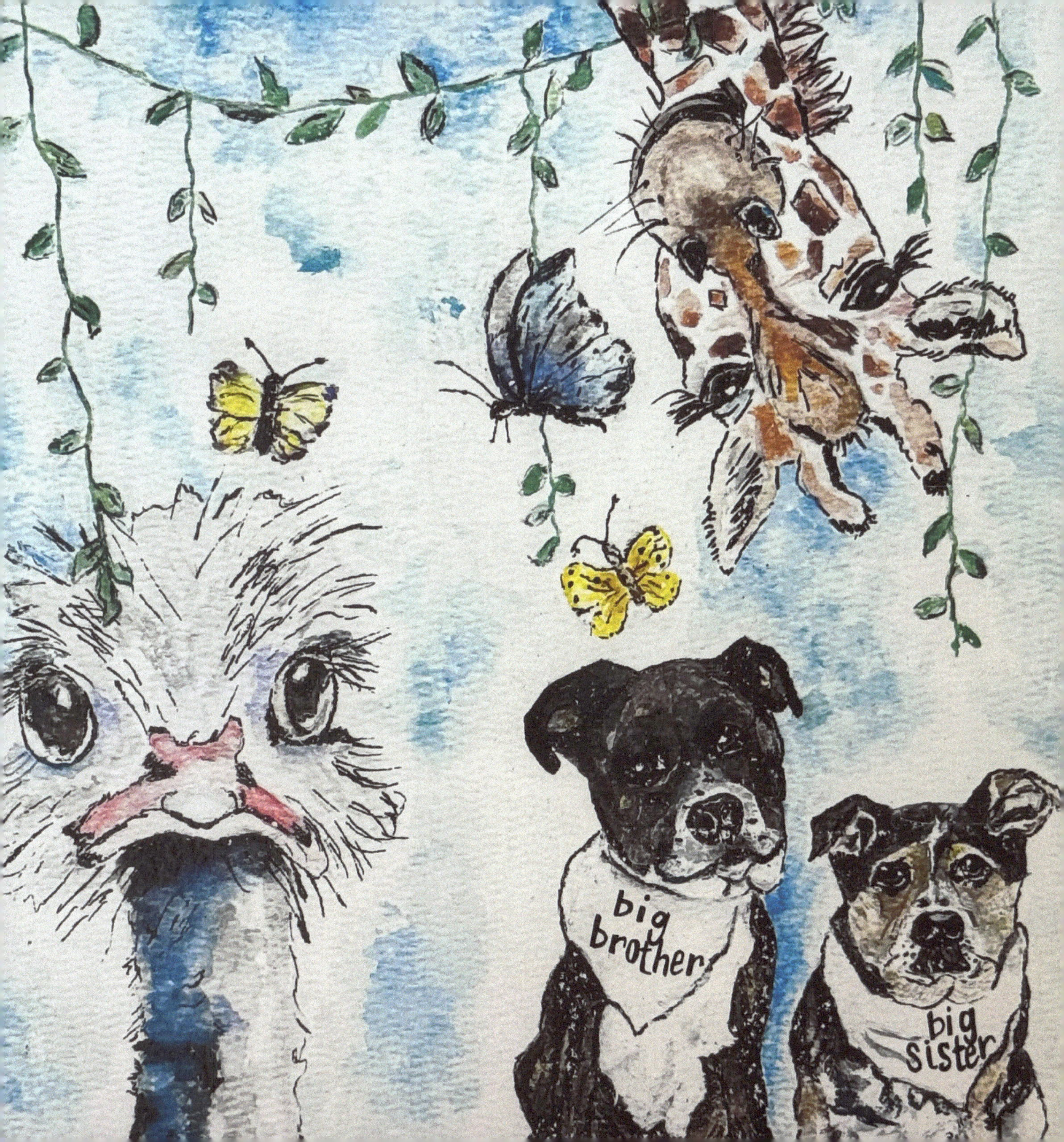

big brother
big sister

Will you be, could you be *Mary Jane* or maybe *Silas Joe?*

At this point, only the Good Lord knows!

Around Weeks 15 to 16, you're sucking your thumb!

Who will you be, and do you know where you came from?

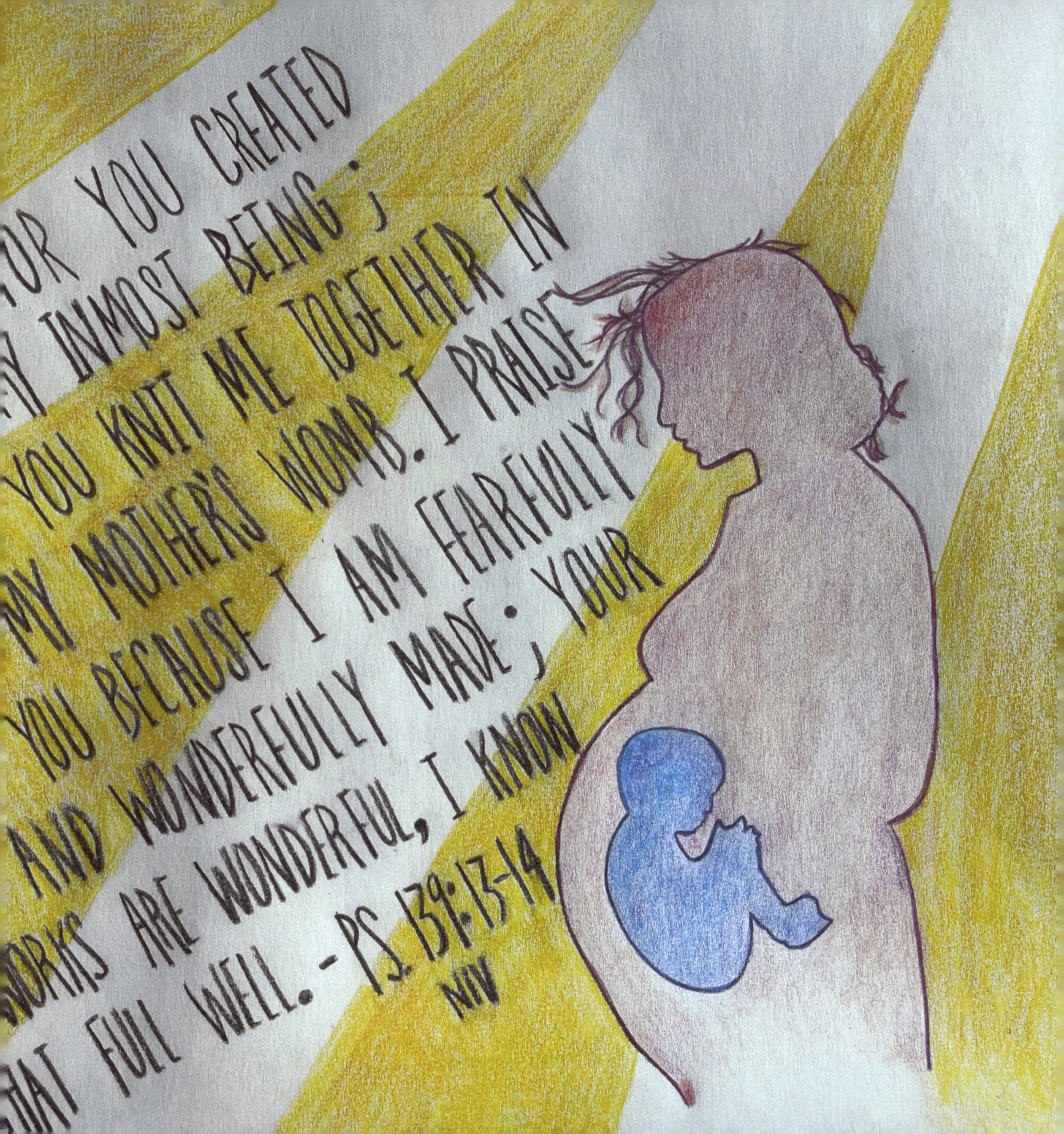
FOR YOU CREATED
MY INMOST BEING;
YOU KNIT ME TOGETHER IN
MY MOTHER'S WOMB. I PRAISE
YOU BECAUSE I AM FEARFULLY
AND WONDERFULLY MADE; YOUR
WORKS ARE WONDERFUL, I KNOW
THAT FULL WELL. - PS. 139:13-14
NIV

Our God the Creator has made you alive.

He has good plans for you and will even help you arrive!

Who will you be? Who will you become?

Will you love music and like the beat of a drum-a-rum-rum?

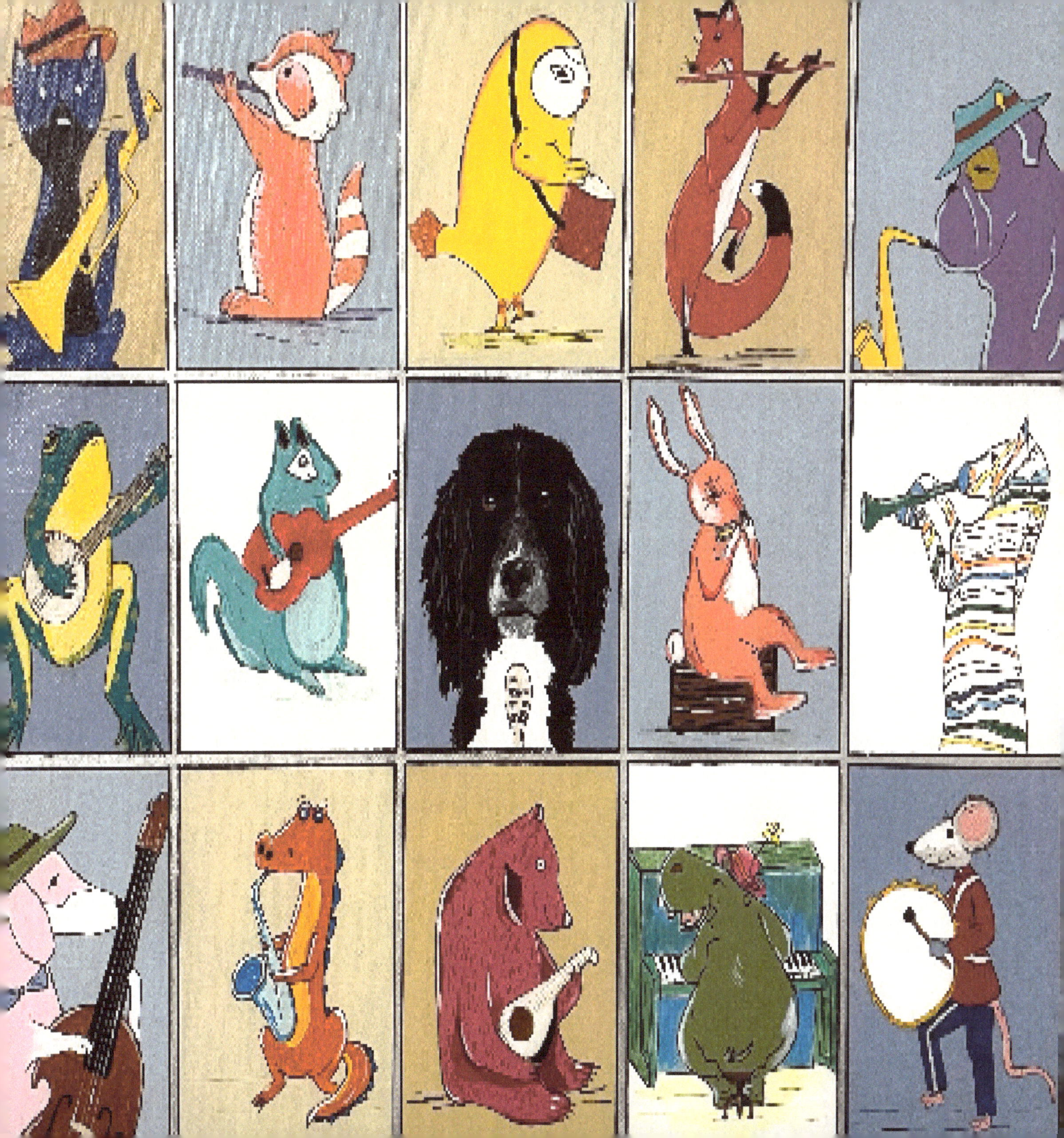

Your eyebrows and eyelashes are growing around Week 22,
You have been chosen, accepted, and that will always be true!
Between Weeks 23 to 24, you can hear noises from outside,
Like music and voices and cars taking people for rides!

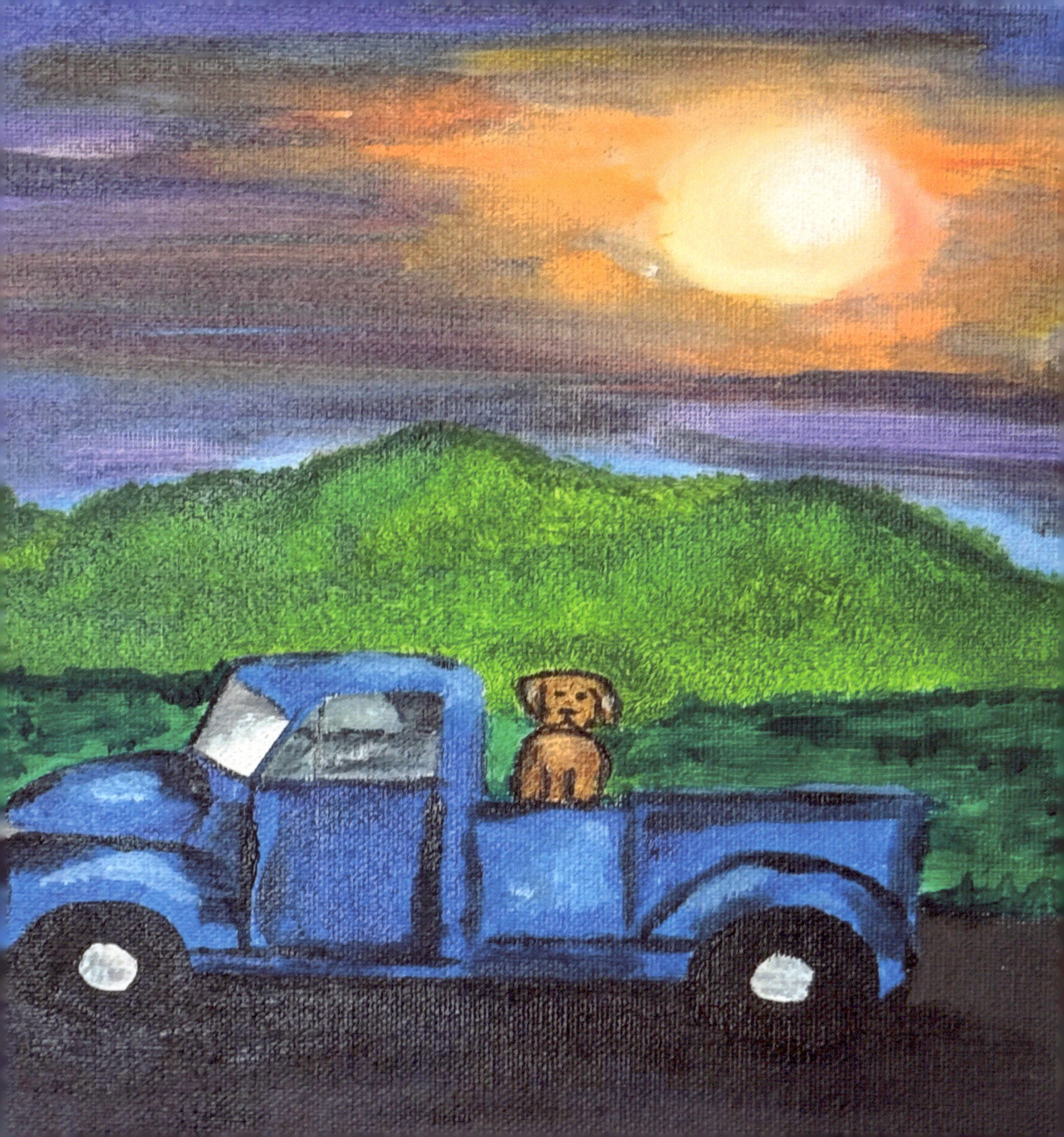

At Week 25, You might have some hair;

I hope you know somehow, you're being covered in prayer!

Will you be a doctor, a teacher, or will you fly planes,

A mommy, a preacher, or will you run trains?

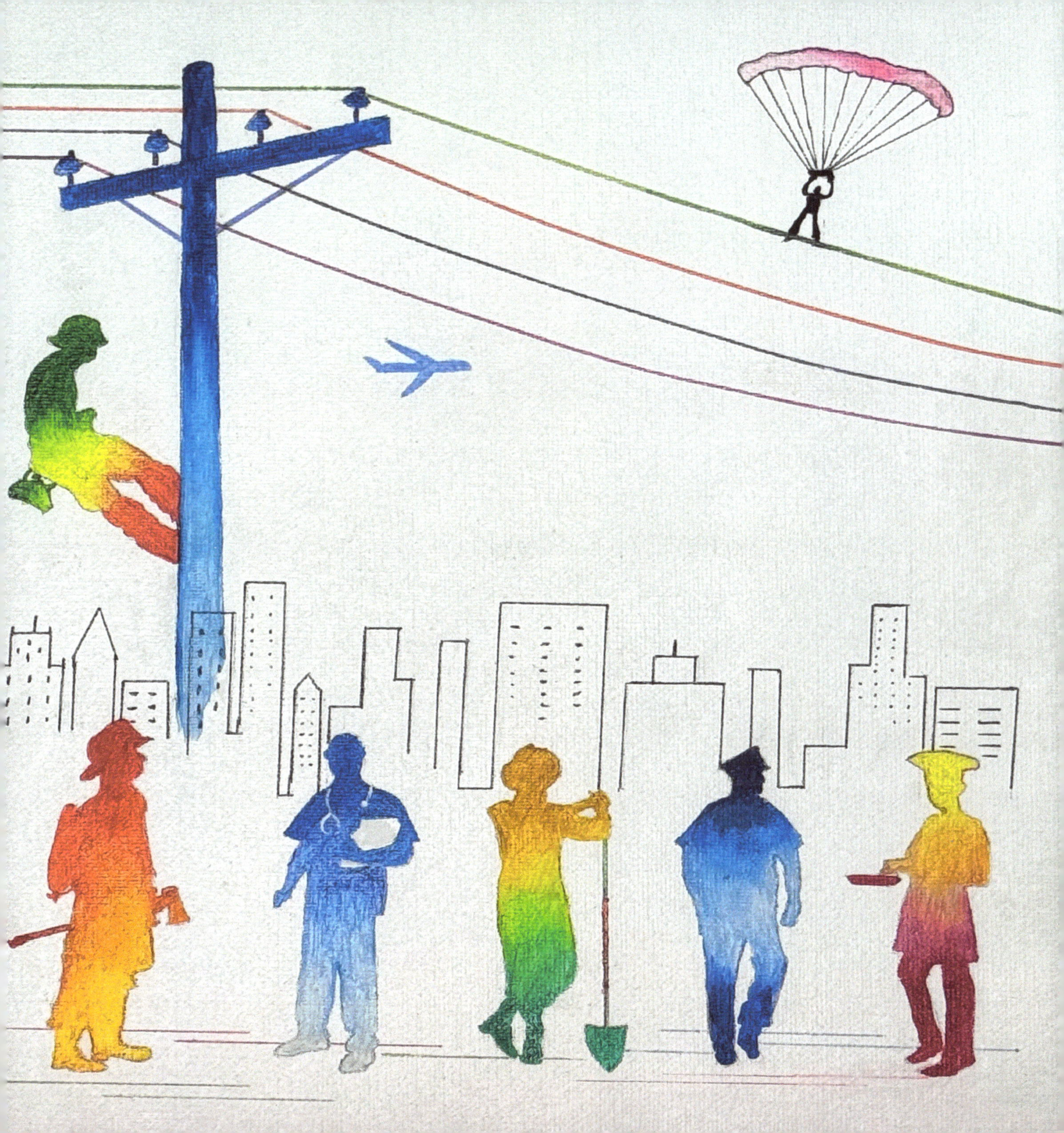

You are God's workmanship, and you'll turn out just fine,
Now, you're starting to sleep & wake at a regular time!
Around Weeks 31 to 32, we'll find you dreaming while you sleep.
Do you chase dogs and butterflies, or are you just counting sheep?

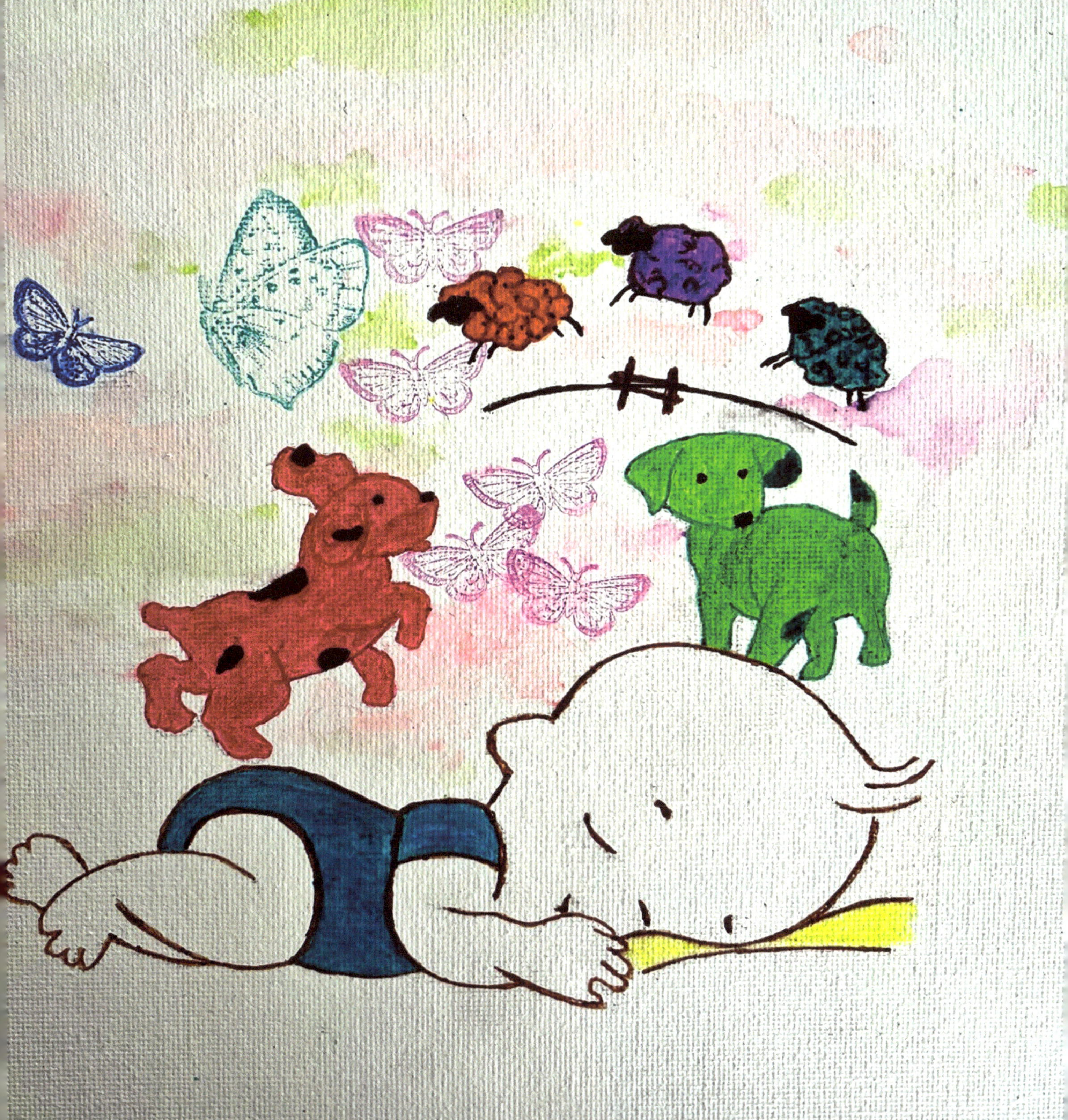

Where you are is probably getting pretty snug,

I can't wait to kiss you all over and give you sweet hugs.

All those that love you can't wait to see

Will you be a "he" or possibly a "she?"

Just so you know, it doesn't matter to me!

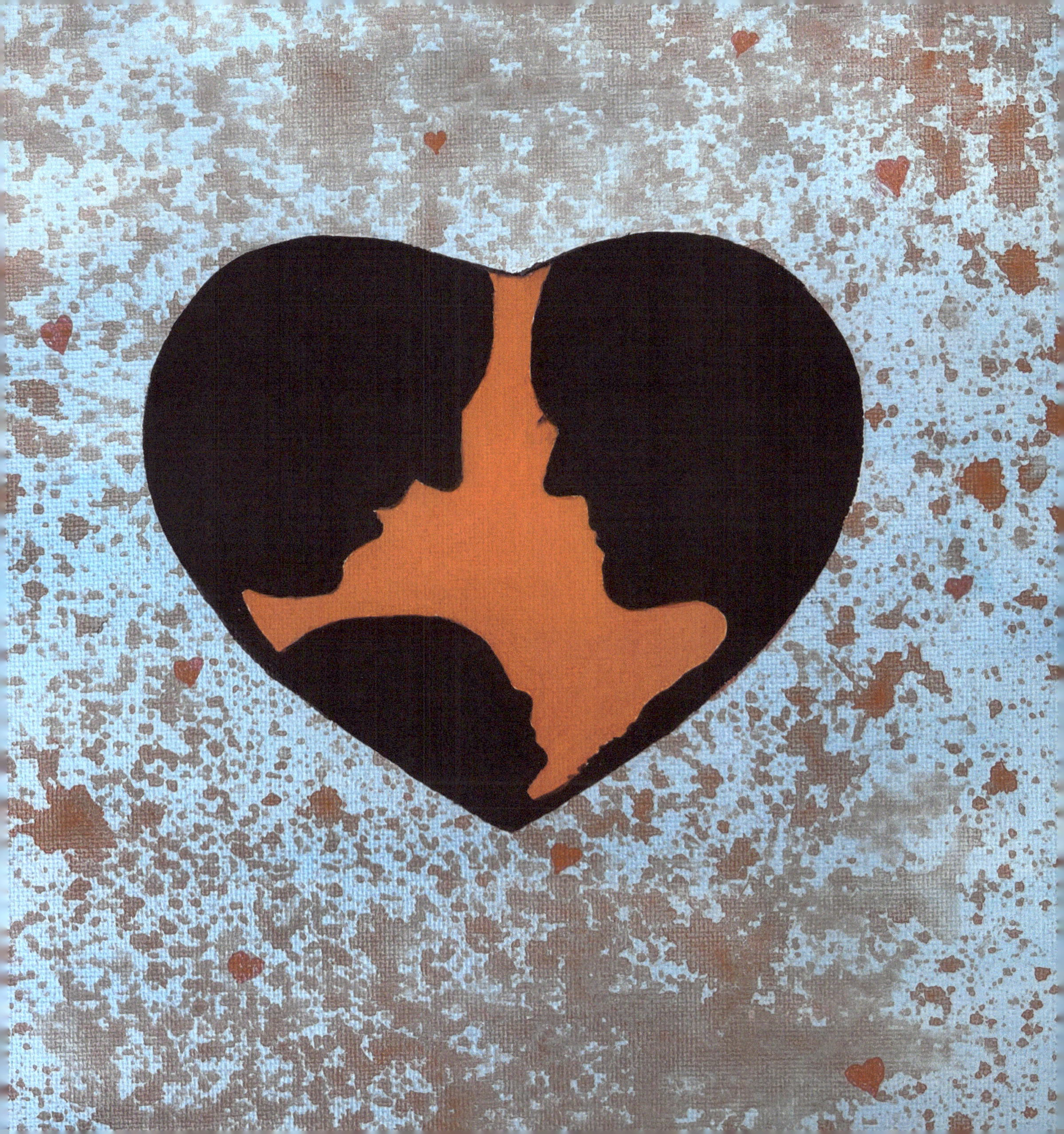

Our God will help shape who you will be,
Smart, kind, honest, confident and free!
You'll be a good friend, helpful and brave
Humble, responsible, and so well-behaved.

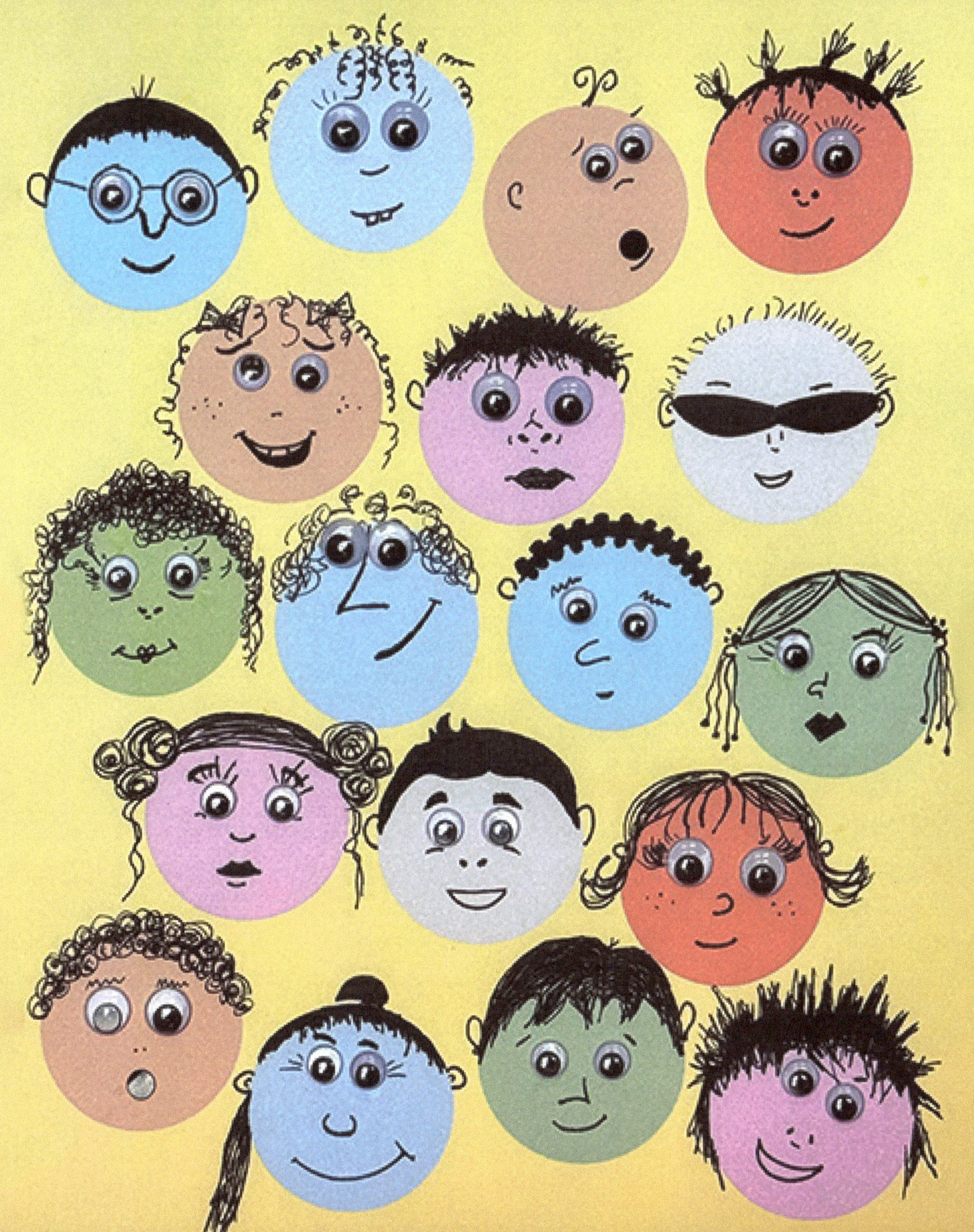

I ask myself over and over, "Who will you be?"
I can't wait to meet you and finally see,
Who you will be, oh, who you will be!

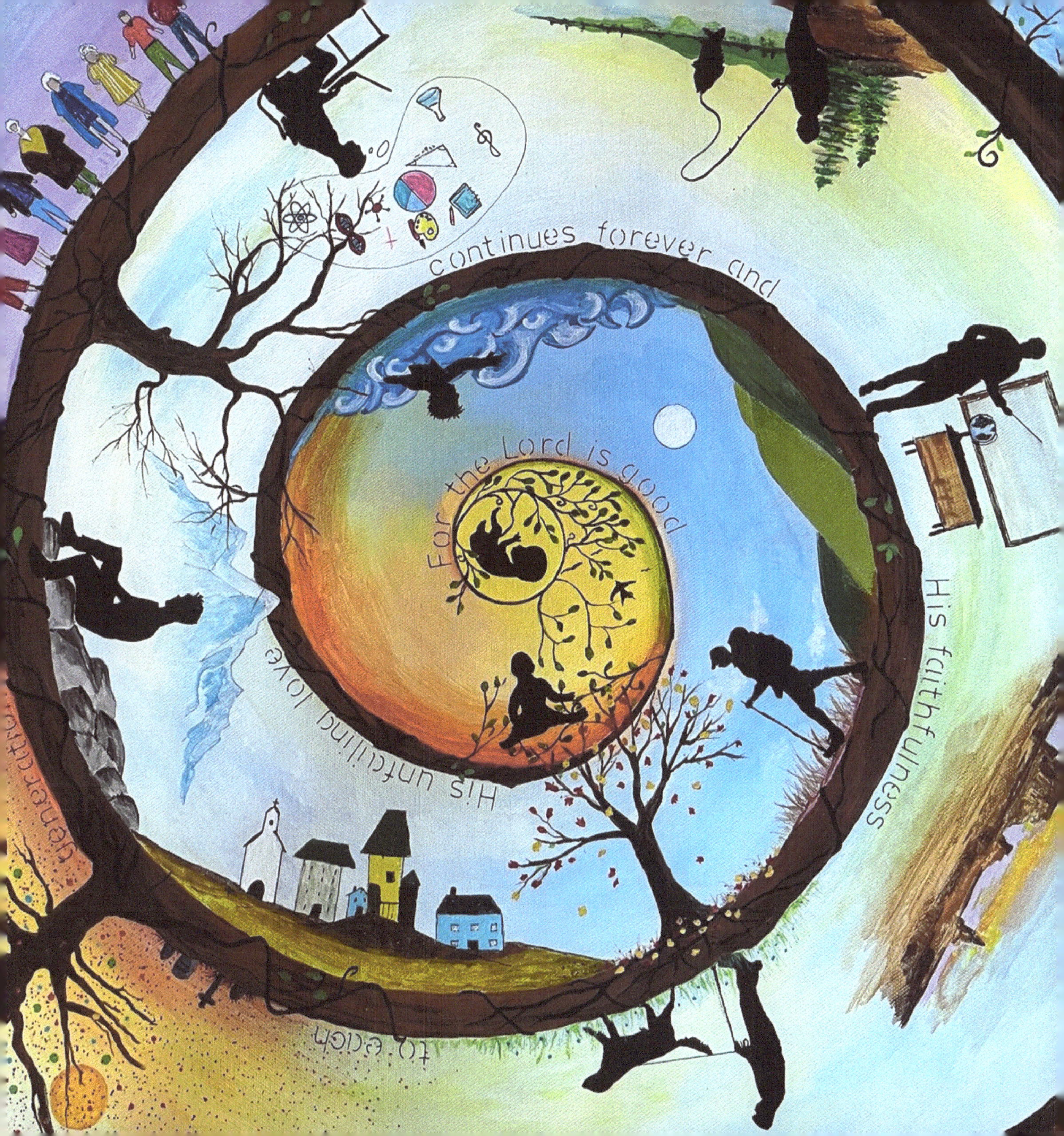

continues forever and
For the Lord is good
His unfailing love
His faithfulness
generation
to each

About the Author

Dawn Barrett is a daughter, sister, wife, mother, and grandmother who loves "words" and enjoys sharing them in forms of encouragement to the people she does life with. Born and raised in the foothills of North Carolina, she has many full-time jobs: pastor's wife, speaker/teacher of women, Eecutive Assistant, Mom and Nana of humans and dogs!

Dawn loves spending time with family, reading, shopping, and watching her talented husband, Joe, complete projects for herself and others!

www.ingramcontent.com/pod-product-compliance
Lightning Source LLC
Chambersburg PA
CBHW040206240726
48664CB00002B/856